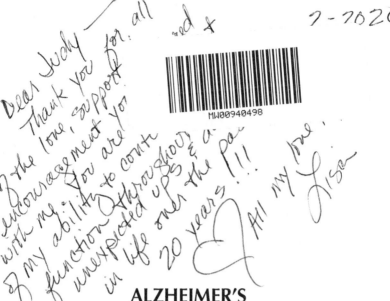

7-2020

Dear Judy —
Thank you for all
the love, support,
encouragement, ...ed
with my ability you are
function throughout
unexpected ups & the pa...
in life over the
20 years !!!
All my love,
Lisa

ALZHEIMER'S
QUICK TIPS FOR CAREGIVERS
Vol. 1: Living With A Wild Raccoon

LISA A. SANTIAGO

outskirts press

Outskirts Press, Inc.
http://www.outskirtspress.com

ISBN: 978-1-4787-9922-1

Lisa A. Santiago
https://www.facebook.com/sadness2smiles/
alz.care.santiago@gmail.com

Front and back covers designed by Kim Tracy
kimtracy52@gmail.com

Author photo credit: Linda Krug
Original photos by Linda Krug and Lisa Santiago

Outskirts Press and the "OP" logo are trademarks belonging to Outskirts Press, Inc.

PRINTED IN THE UNITED STATES OF AMERICA

DEDICATION – To my grandma...

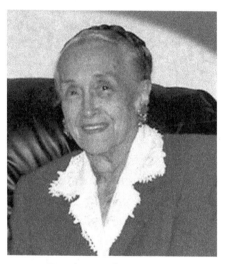

Bessie Marie Dugena

Sitting quietly in a rare moment of peace, you might ask, "What's my purpose?" No matter what you've achieved, the answer can seem insignificant. In these moments, it's helpful to consider the domino effect that your choices will have on everyone around you. My grandma is my best example of the power of this domino effect. Her choices touched many people in ways that she never would have imagined.

Over the years, Grandma shared many memories of

her life. She lived through some horrible experiences. It was easy to see that she could have grown into a bitter and spiteful person, but she chose a better path. Instead of blaming others for hard times or unfair outcomes, she viewed sad events as lessons to make us more resilient.

Many times, she told me that she wasn't perfect - that she made mistakes. To repay whatever mistakes she thought she made, Grandma chose to use her life experiences to help others become resilient and independent as well. Some of those choices had a domino effect that impacted my life.

Thanks to Grandma's loving interventions and consistent support to my parents, my sister and I did not become part of the sad statistics of inner-city children born to teen parents. My parents worked very hard to give us a better life than they had, but the extra support and advice from my grandma played a big role in allowing us to live in crime-free neighborhoods and attend high-ranking schools.

Grandma taught me many things (how to crochet, needlepoint, read a pattern and use a sewing machine). She also gave me a couple gifts of which even family members are unaware. First is the gift of a spanking! From this, I learned that anyone who pours soda on her sister's bed is going to get a good spanking. Lesson learned – food or drink in bed is asking for all sorts of trouble! And second, she gave me the gift of seeing adventure and opportunity instead of fear. When I had my first opportunity to study abroad, I had only half of the mandatory down-payment. I thought it was a sign that I was not supposed to go. I discussed it with my grandma. She thought I was afraid and she was right – I had never left the country or traveled so far alone. I didn't ask her for it but my grandma offered me a loan to cover the rest of the down-payment. Thanks to Grandma's support and encouragement I was able to study art and design in Japan. All that I learned was priceless!

Many people and other variables helped turn my big dreams into accomplishments, but going back in time – going back to years before I was born - it's clear to see that key components of success began with my grandma's love for her children, her adventurous spirit, and her life-long support for teaching and education.

When you ask "What's my purpose?", know that your choices will have a domino effect that can impact future generations in ways that you cannot imagine.

In these books, Grandma's spirit lives on in ways that she never could have imagined. Her life and experiences can continue to help people - inspiring smiles, joy, and happiness. This is the domino effect of her life!

Table of Contents

Preface

Question: Why write this book?

Answer: While working in an adult psychiatric unit, I saw many individuals whose mental illnesses hindered their abilities to function in everyday life. I became familiar with the systems put in place to help them. In addition to this, as a college-level psychology instructor, I keep up with advances in brain and memory research in order to share this with my students. All of this knowledge and first-hand experience dealing with the brain and mental illnesses led me to believe that I was prepared to easily care for my grandma as Alzheimer's tried to take her further and further away. It only took a few months for me to learn that I was wrong! I needed more options. I needed more solutions.

How it began...
I moved to Iowa in the 1980s to work with medical students at the University of Iowa. Living in Iowa

allowed me to regularly visit my grandma in her home in Cedar Rapids. Years passed with both good and sad times. Two of the saddest times include being with her as her last love passed away in the home they shared for over 30 years, and taking her to have a toe amputated from diabetes complications. After this surgery, her balance was hindered enough that she was at risk of falling with every step. Her refusal to use a walker did not help that problem at all. (Tip #5 helps address this common problem.) With each traumatic loss, she was able to do less and less. Eventually, I was visiting every weekend to do her grocery shopping and laundry.

During my weekly visits, if she was in an ornery mood, she'd say, "I hope you're not doing this because you think you'll be in my will. I have too many grandchildren to give everyone something. I have five children and all my money is being split-up between them equally. I expect your parents to take care of you. That's not my job. So if you're here for money, you'd better forget it!" I told her that I knew I was not getting any money and I was there because I loved her. That silly answer clearly irritated her. She'd purse her lips, roll her eyes and then change the subject.

Grandma was feisty and fiercely independent. As a teenager during World War II, a particular graphic image had a huge impact on her life. That image was of *Rosie the Riveter* (on a poster for Westinghouse Electric Corporation). You know this image when you see it – Rosie's gorgeous brunette curls are tied-up in a red scarf with white polka-dots. On a bright yellow background, we see her arm raised to show us her fist and a beautifully firm bi-cep. The text on the poster proudly declares to all women, "We can do it."

This image showed Grandma that women can be beautiful and powerful on their own. With her gorgeous brunette curls and feminine but solid physical features, this graphic image of Rosie very much resembled my grandma in her 20s. Rosie and my grandma looked similar enough that they could have been sisters.

Art History 101 Refresher...

Having a Master's Degree in Art Education, I am compelled to share this valuable piece of art and history with you. It's the power of the domino effect (noted in the dedication). We never know what will happen when we share valid information. Maybe this will inspire you – remind you that "You can do it." I have this image hanging in my kitchen

---

for just that reason!

- In the 1940s, *Rosie the Riveter* presented a strong female image that had not been socially promoted in the US before. For the first time in American history, Rosie offered young women another option – they didn't have to get married and stay home to raise children – they could get a job, earn their own money and be independent.

- This is a truly fascinating piece of history. If you're interested, there are also other versions of Rosie which are fun to see and read about on the History.com website. The direct web link can be found in the reference list at the end of this book. If you don't like to read, don't worry. There are also short informative videos in addition to the text and photos.

These were the formative years of Grandma's life and society was changing in drastic ways. Men were being sent off to war and, for the first time, rather than stay home to cook and clean in dresses and high heels, women were being highly recruited to work for the war efforts. The recruitment efforts focused on placing women in factory jobs where they would use power tools and run industrial machines rather than sit behind desks to type memos and answer phones. When we understand this history, it's no wonder that Rosie became my grandma's number one role model. Considering the current population of people in their 70s, 80s, and 90s, it's quite possible that the social changes of this era played a huge role for your loved one as well.

By all of her accounts, my grandma's home life included a great deal of verbal and physical abuse. This may have been why Grandma was ahead of her time in her efforts to be free and independent. It may have been the reason why she saw sad and unfair events as the keys to teaching resilience. With Rosie plastered everywhere as a role model for female strength and independence, as a teenager, my grandma decided to run away from her abusive home-life. She hopped on a train headed to California. Upon arrival, she planned to become "Bessie the Riveter."

Grandma shared this story many times. It was one of my favorites, but no matter how many times she told it, she always looked stunned when she got to the part where she was "busted" in Colorado and forced by police to go back home. She said she was so scared to go back that she begged them to put her in a foster home instead!

Sadly, the immense power of her independent spirit

could not stop the arrival of Alzheimer's and years of life when she could never be home alone again.

The 100-Year Flood…

The biggest problems began in 2008 when the "100-Year Flood" devastated portions of the Midwestern United States. Grandma worked hard and planned well for an independent life after her retirement, but this flood took it all away. She lost her home, her rental property, and her souvenir shop in Czech Village - a hobby that was to be her "happy place" until the very end.

To help explain traumatic events, we often hear phrases such as, "You had to be there.", or "You never know what you'll do until it happens to you." This disaster is one of those events. For thousands of people, life was forever changed.

We usually think of water as a cleansing agent; fresh, pure, reviving and renewing. In a flood like this, water becomes a deadly assassin. There is no favoritism - no mercy for life or love. Everything is destroyed – including the air!

You might be wondering, "How is it possible for air to be destroyed?" To help grasp the realities of this type of disaster, try to remember the smell of damp dirty items that were left balled-up in a hamper or in a gym bag for a few days. That smell can make the strongest of men gag. It's hard to believe, but for months, the smell of this entire city was worse than that ghastly smell!

When the rain finally stops, everyone waits for the waters to subside. It takes weeks. From floor to ceiling, everything is soaked and covered in a sticky, mud-like, black smelly sludge. It's a serious health hazard. For those who don't realize the dangers, there are federal and state agents on the street corners encouraging all clean-up workers and volunteers to get a free tetanus shot. They hand out white hazmat suits, face masks, and plastic gloves. They tell you to put them on before you touch or move anything. Your brain wants to pretend that you're on a movie set for a horror movie. For a millisecond you think, "Maybe I don't really need to wear that mask or gloves." but the dangers are real, and you follow the rules.

When the police barriers are down and you are finally allowed back to your property, there is hope. In the clean-up, family and friends help to sift through belongings with a goal of finding even one cherished item: a ring handed down over generations, a photo of someone no longer on this earth, or the key to a safety deposit box. As the hours go by you realize that the search for specific items is hopeless and then you try to save anything that can be safely cleaned: a ceramic coffee mug, a stainless steel pot, or even a plastic flower pot. You need something to prove that your time was not wasted – something to prove that all you worked for has not been lost.

In this photo, Grandma is sitting outside of her shop, trying to save as much as she could.

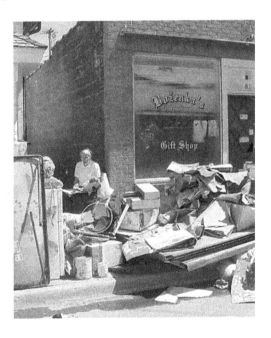

The losses from this flood sent Grandma's Alzheimer's symptoms into overdrive. By her standards, she was homeless – she had no home of her own. Amazingly, she managed to stay positive. I never heard her cry or complain. Instead, she told everyone, "I'm happy that I got out with my cat and my favorite denim skirt."

With big hearts and good intentions, various family members opened their homes and tried to take care of her. Within weeks or months, the stress took its toll on each of them and she was bounced to someone else. I reminded everyone of my training and said I wanted her to live with me. No one cared about that stuff. They said I was too young or that I had too many jobs to care for her. They said that they were retired, "Home all the time" so it would be easy for them and better for her.

No more moving from home to home...

After two years of Grandma moving from family member to family member, the last option was exhausted. Bouncing - sometimes across state lines - from home to home was over. With less than eight hours of notice, she was brought to my house with all of her belongings in giant black garbage bags. The drop-off was quick. There was both guilt and relief on the faces of those who left her. For everyone, the emotions were complex and confusing, but Grandma was finally with me full-time.

Relieved and excited, I unpacked the black bags and did all I could to help her feel comfortable. There would be changes to everyday life, but I was committed to repaying her for the things she gave to my parents. The tangible and emotional support she gave them allowed me, and my sister, to have opportunities in life that we would never have had otherwise. That truth was always at the forefront of my mind.

I was certain that I had the academic and practical working knowledge to meet all of her needs. To my surprise, my books and work experiences had not given me all I needed to manage the Alzheimer's disease with the ease I had anticipated. There were many moments when I was shocked by Grandma's thoughts, actions, and behaviors.

Love is not enough...

With a concept similar to the famous saying, 'Give a man a fish and he will eat for a day. Teach a man to fish and he will eat for his lifetime.' this book is the result of being taught how to fish for what I needed. Things happened that were not in a textbook and I began to fully realize why <u>love is simply not enough to be a full-time caregiver in your home</u>. I understood why my family members had to "give up." Thanks to my academic background and professional experiences, I was able to develop practical solutions to solve the problems that make many caregivers sad, angry, and frustrated.

Tips for everyone who needs them – This is a book for the masses...

As Alzheimer's disease continues to increase in our population at a devastating rate, <u>this book is written for a mass public audience.</u> The goal of these three volumes is to help provide caregivers quick and easy solutions to some of the most common problems. The solutions provided here are based on both personal experience and research. With this in mind, I have tried to avoid crossing the line into advanced academic writing that can be difficult to read, but I have included some academic tidbits and easy-to-find references for those who want to delve deeper into these topics without having to read complex statistical data in research journal articles.

As a caregiver, if you're reading this, you know the feelings of frustration, fear, guilt, and helplessness that are part of your "new normal". You also know the joy you feel when your loved one has moments of clarity - the moments that keep you going and praying for one more good day or just another good hour.

This book is for you, the caregiver. I want to give you all of my fish and share the tips for catching them!

Sending you love and hugs for all you are doing,

~ Lisa A. Santiago

Acknowledgments

First and foremost, I must thank my entire family for all of the love and support they have given me in my lifetime. I would not be who I am without my parents, Paul, Joanie, and JoAnne, cheering me on (and sometimes giving a needed swift kick in the behind) in order to move forward through life's most painful and difficult lessons. They made me who I am. They taught me to survive and find success without stepping on other people to get there.

Thanks to my aunts Marianne and Betty Anne who both took time away from their own busy lives to help me care for my grandma. Marianne, with her good friend Michael, used many vacation days to sweep grandma away for weekend adventures at nearby casinos. This provided me a few days to reenergize. My aunt Betty Anne would visit frequently with my cousin Debbie. With every visit, they brought gifts for Grandma, made us a healthy lunch, and shared family updates.

Much thanks to my uncle Freddy who often worked as a free chauffeur, transporting my grandma back and forth from Iowa to Chicago and back again. Throughout the years he and his wife Judi sent many thoughtful and gorgeous gifts, such as Ugg slippers and pearl bracelets. After Grandma lost everything in the flood of 2008 she was thankful for anything, but these very special gifts reminded her that she was cherished. She knew these were extra-special and she felt as pampered as a queen every day.

Another "Thank you" to the Gary Howard and Dan Krug families for inviting me and my grandma to join in the many holiday and family events over the years that she was with us. She loved the food, games, and entertainment. In these homes, she always felt welcomed and safe.

Finally, big hugs and thanks to my personal critique team. They critiqued numerous drafts of this book and helped to make this first volume a piece of reading that everyone could enjoy. This book would not be nearly as wonderful without the input and suggestions from Charles Burm, Eric Dimalanta, and Ranelle Downey.

These gifts of time, love, and energy are things that no amount of money can buy. I am forever grateful.

Understand Your Motives
- Not Everyone Can, or
Should, be a Caregiver!

THERE IS NO need to add guilt to an already bad or sad situation. The more clearly you understand your motives, the more peace and calm you will have on a daily basis. This section addresses some of the main reasons that people choose to be caregivers and provides some additional thoughts to consider before you take on this challenging role.

If you have already taken on the role, but feel more frustrated than fulfilled, I encourage you to review this section. You may have taken on this role without considering the long-term domino effect on your life. You may or may not choose to change the current living arrangements but if you understand your initial motives, it might bring you some much needed internal peace.

MONEY: Are you trying to save money?

Are you trying to save your loved one's money?

What was the goal when your loved one saved money for retirement and old age? Was it to have money to live well until the end or was it saved as an inheritance gift for you?

Would your loved one want to use his or her life-savings for in-home private assistance?

Would your loved one want to use his or her money to rent a room or apartment in a senior living facility? Why or why not?

Be cautious when money is a key factor in your decision to be a full-time caregiver in your home.

Your long-term health and sanity are more valuable than money.

LOVE and TRUST: Are you the only person who can provide quality care?

Clearly evaluate the needs of your loved one. Are you ready to make needed adjustments without concern for "how it looks?" or "not matching your style?"

Are you willing to clean urine-soaked clothing and bedding if needed?

Are you comfortable touching your loved one if you have to bathe him or her? Will you be comfortable putting lotion or needed medication on his or her feet or other body parts if needed? If there's an "accident" in the middle of your day, or right before you're walking out of the house, can you clean-up the mess with kindness and understanding or will you get angry?

Eventually you will need safety rails, ramps, motion censored lights, and alarms. You'll probably need to add locks or other types of deterrents on cabinets, refrigerators, and freezers. There is a lot to consider in providing quality care. Safety is key at all times and this can be tricky. It's a bit more complicated than the demands of restricting a toddler or new puppy to a room that we know we have outfitted for safety. In our case, we are dealing with a full-grown adult. This full-grown adult has a lifetime of knowledge and awareness that comes and goes without any warning. When we are not in the room with this beloved full-grown adult, anything can happen. A baby gate placed in a doorway for protection can turn into a hazard – it can pinch fingers or lead to a fall. Our fully grown loved one can get into things and places that a child or puppy could never reach. Our fully grown loved one is capable of moving or dismantling safety gadgets and barriers. All of these issues must be considered, expected, and planned for.

RELATIONSHIP and HISTORY: Are you moving from a lifetime of receiving care to giving it?

For me, this was easy to understand and handle. Grandma always had her own life, jobs, and responsibilities. In my life, my grandma was never my full-time caregiver. She didn't change my diapers or take me to the hospital for medical emergencies. It was not a habit for my sister and I to be with her over-night or for weekends. She did not bathe me or read me stories at bedtime. When I was growing up, Grandma made it clear that she was not a free babysitting service. She always lived nearby, but she was not with us every day.

My grandma was always "old" to me. When I was 5 and she was 45, to me, that was already ancient. As far back as I can remember Grandma was always the slowest. She was slower than my parents, slower than my aunts and uncles and definitely slower than I was. In our entire existence, this fact remained the same: Grandma was slower and older than I was. Over the years, seeing the declines in her mental and physical state was difficult because I could see how much it made her sad, but when a child sees those declines in a parent – that can cause a big rip in the fabric of your view of life. The change in world-view is not the same as when a grandchild sees these declines in a grandparent. Grandparents were always slower, now, they are even more slow than before. It's not a huge change in our view of life and aging processes.

There are added emotional strains if you are caring for your parents or your cohort siblings rather than a grandparent. Our parents have been our teachers, leaders, and guides. With the exception of those hormonal and rebellious teen years, we knew our parents were smarter and stronger. It was their job to protect and care for us. Watching their decline is a sadness that some people do not handle very well. Often, the frustrations of repeating simple instructions or directions can lead to yelling, insults, or name-calling and that is emotional abuse.

As the child who has now turned into a caregiver, there are a variety of reasons why the frustration can turn to anger. This is an emotionally twisted, complex, and sad reality that I have seen in action many times. If you try to be conscious of this, and pause when you begin to feel angry, you can work to avoid this negative outcome if you want to. It's not easy, but you can do it. Hopefully the tips in these volumes will help you to minimize, or completely eliminate, these frustrating times.

If you are caring for a cohort sibling (a brother or sister

in your own age group), witnessing these declines can be paralyzing. There is likely to be a moment when you think, "This could be me", or "I'm next." That reality can take your breath away. It might begin to lead your mind into dark and scary places. You need to be prepared and remember that it's not happening to you. There are many more factors, beyond genetics alone, which lead to disease and illness. You and your sibling made different decisions in life and now, you are choosing to be the caregiver.

Attending support group meetings can help to handle some of these problems. You can usually find them through your local hospital or hospice centers. Many of these support groups can be joined for free. If you want individualized help, you might be happier with the services of a certified therapist, social worker, or a life coach who can privately assist and support you as needed. If you're embarrassed, or don't have time to drive to an office, some certified professionals, including myself, are able and willing to conduct all sessions over the phone.

BUILD MEMORIES and MAKE UP FOR LOST TIME: Do you want quality time that you never had or are you trying to make up for lost time before it's too late?

Yes, you can build memories for yourself. You may be able to alleviate or heal some old wounds from days gone by, but know that the moments of clarity, sharing, and healing are only momentary for your loved one. It is very likely that he or she will not remember your deep heartfelt conversations tomorrow. You need to be okay with that. You can be okay (not have your feelings hurt) if you remember that you are doing this to heal your own wounds. You are doing this for your own long-term peace of mind. You don't want to regret that you never said, "I'm sorry." or "I love you." Remember that you are doing this <u>to create and build **your** memories</u>. If you can do this, you can still feel good when your loved one doesn't remember any of it later.

Your loved one does not have to live with you in order to build memories. There are other living arrangement options. They may not be desired options, but there are always other options. Other options commonly include:

- your loved one living with another family member
- your loved one living with one of his or her friends
- your loved one living in a nursing home
- your loved one living at home with paid help until the very last dollar of savings is gone
- your loved one living in a facility supported by local, state, or federal funds

These options might not feel good to you. They may

not be what you want, but they are viable options. When you remember this, the demands of this role are easier to handle. This is directly related to the perception of control discussed in Tip #4. It's a powerful concept that we can all use to feel better about almost anything. Remind yourself *why* you chose to have your loved one with you and then remember that you can make a different choice at any time.

Another common reason that people take on this role is because they feel that they are running out or time. Maybe you have plenty of childhood memories, but other priorities took over as adult life moved forward. Now, it feels as if time is running out and you want to make up for that lost time before it's too late. If you squeeze in full-time caregiving during the last years of life, will this help you gain the quality moments that you desire? Will you have to give-up, trade, or minimize time on other things in order to find the hours needed for quality time with your loved one? Only you can answer those questions honestly.

For people who have children, it's impossible to imagine that there could be a time when you will not recognize them, but Alzheimer's can take these pieces of personal history away. It has nothing to do with you or how much love, care, and devotion was shared between you and this loved one. This is not about you. It's a terrible illness that removes memories of all types. As yet, research on brains and memories has no definitive answers to explain why some core elements of life and love disappear when Alzheimer's strikes. Taking care of your loved one may or may not inspire happy flashes of memory. If you take on this role expecting memories of children or grandchildren to come rushing back into the mind of your loved one, you may be disappointed.

There were many days that my grandma could not remember how many children she had. Even if she remembered that she had five children, if asked for their names, she could not remember all of them. Often, she thought I was one of her daughters. I did not correct her. Those types of constant corrections can lead to irritation for everyone. They can also make your loved one feel sad as he or she is forced to realize these errors. It's not worth it. It made no difference if I was Lisa, Marianne or JoAnne. Grandma knew she was with a family member who cared for her and that's all that mattered.

When your elderly loved one does not remember key life relationships such as this, it is usually one of the most painful and confusing issues to handle. It's best to expect this as the disease takes over. In the next section, Tip # 1 provides some simple steps to help minimize this problem.

Mini Photo Album Reinforces Knowledge of Relationships

ONE OF THE most heartbreaking events for people caring for a loved one suffering from Alzheimer's or dementia is witnessing the inability of a loved one to recognize the people that he or she loved the most. In time, parents may no longer recognize their children or grandchildren. This is something that is impossible for most people to imagine, and then you see it happen before your very eyes.

Here is a simple tool to help ease this problem:

1. Buy a cheap mini plastic photo album - the kind that holds about a dozen 4x6 photos. Finding a plastic photo album is important

because it will need to be wiped clean fairly often. Most of these little plastic photo albums allow for a photo to be slipped into the cover. (I bought this one - shown in the following photo - at Walmart for under $3.00. I've also seen them at the Dollar Tree and at Target.) If you use one that does not allow the option to slide your own photo into the cover, choose one with a very plain light-colored cover so that you can print your loved one's name on it. Choosing a light colored cover will make your printed words easier to see and read. The cover must quickly and easily grab the attention of your loved one!

2. On the cover, place a photo of your loved one. With a black permanent marker, **print** his or her name on it. As shown in the example, my grandma's cover had her photo. On a Post-It note that was cut to fit, you can clearly read, "Bessie's Photos" – this was very helpful in getting her attention. Every morning, when she saw this on the kitchen table she would say, "Oh, that's me. This is mine!" and then she would begin to flip through it.

3. Print color photos of all the people your loved one sees or talks to on a regular basis.

4. Try to use photos of your loved one <u>with</u> the person they see or talk to on a regular basis.

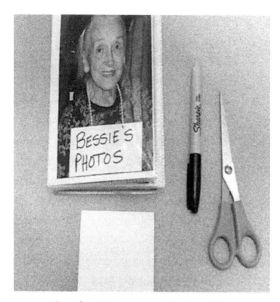

Simple & Inexpensive Supplies

5. Use a black permanent marker to print the name or relationship of each person in the photo.

   » I advise writing on the Post-It note rather than writing on the photo or plastic cover. It's a time saver. You can correct mistakes much more easily by simply writing on a new Post-It and placing it where you need it. If you choose to write on the photo, you must let the ink dry before you place the photo into the plastic sleeve. If you are not patient, the wet ink smears on both the photo and the plastic sleeve. I ruined some photos this way. If you choose to write on the plastic sleeve (which I also tried), as you wipe and clean these pages over time, the permanent ink gets wiped off along with sticky fingerprints.

» Since we had a few pets, I also included photos of each pet and wrote the pets name on the photo. My grandma would look at the photo and say, "Oh, that's this one right here." When she said this, she was pointing to our German shepherd Frankie. Frankie was always by Grandma's side. (In Volume III, I'll review the research on the emotional gifts that furry family members provide and share more about how Frankie guarded and protected Grandma till the very end!)

Include pets - EXAMPLE:

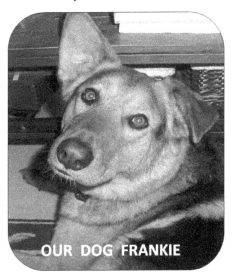

OUR DOG FRANKIE

*** *Use keywords that provide ownership such as "our house", "your firstborn son", "Bessie's cat", etc. This will help your loved one feel connection and belongingness.*

Your loved one can look at the photos and read the relationship and the names of people, places, pets – anything that is common to see every day. Reviewing these photos and reading the key pieces of relationships will help your loved one feel safe and loved.

6. Keep this mini photo album handy. I kept Grandma's on the kitchen table. Look at these photos (together with your loved one) every day, at every meal. Ask your loved one to read the names and relationships to you. In addition to helping save some key memories, this event can also inspire some fun conversations about friends and family!

7. When someone calls to talk to your loved one, open the photo album to a photo of the person on the phone. Show the photo and say, "This is the person on the phone for you. It's your _____." Show your loved one the photo as he/she is engaging with the caller.

8. When someone visits, show your loved one a photo of him/herself with that visitor and read the relationship. For example, "This is your good friend from church. Here is a picture of you with her last year." These cues help to

> reduce the fear, anxiety, and stress from what is likely to be the first question asked, which is - "Do you remember me?"

By showing the photo, you have evidence that there is a happy and long-standing relationship that can be trusted. By explaining who this visitor is, you remove the stress of your loved one trying very hard to remember. Asking your loved one, "Do you know who this is?" may seem like a simple question. Many people believe that the longer the relationship lasted, the easier it should be to remember, but none of these expectations match what often happens in real life. For someone with Alzheimer's, this seemingly simple question may be impossible to answer.

Avoid the stress that comes with this type of questioning. Always announce who the visitor is and what the relationship is. Show photos as valid proof whenever possible.

Avoid discussions that reference the recent past such as, "What have you done this week?", "What did you eat today?", or "Do you remember..." Instead, focus on the current moment such as, "Are you comfortable?" or "Are you hungry?"

During the visit, do something that can be enjoyed together in the moment such as playing a card or board game. My grandma loved to play *Scrabble* or

UpWords. We played either one of those games every weekend. To simplify the rules, we decided that the person with the least tiles at the end of the game was the winner. These decisions are within your control. Change what you need to change to keep these activities simple and fun! The greatest thing to hear from your loved one is, "Let's play another game!" There were weekends when Grandma and I would play these games for two hours!

- *Helpful hint: This suggestion is based on a real-life event when Grandma's first photo album fell out while transporting the walker into the trunk of a friend's car. Make at least 3 identical mini-photo albums. Keep one on the kitchen table, one in the bag on your loved one's walker, and one as a "back-up" for the day that one of these gets misplaced.*

TIP **2**

Brain Cells Can Regenerate - Kale is a Brain Power Veggie!

It was once believed that when brain cells died, that was it; whatever those cells controlled was gone forever. Today we know this is not necessarily the case. Recent studies confirm that our brains can regenerate cells and create new neural connections throughout our lifetime. Current science refers to this as brain plasticity, neural plasticity, or neural regeneration.

Teaching college-level psychology courses requires me to keep up with current research. The concept of brain plasticity is something I teach in all of my courses. At a conference in Iowa City, Iowa, I learned something truly new and fascinating. I learned that diet and nutrition could also help improve my grandma's short-term memory.

At this conference, I saw a life-changing presentation by Dr. Terry Wahls who was diagnosed with progressive multiple sclerosis (MS). As the disease took over, she was eventually confined to a wheelchair. Dr. Wahls feared that she would be restricted from practicing clinical medicine. She shared that, as a scientist and physician, she had access to the "best and most current" medications. She also shared that these "best and most current" drugs made her feel worse. She showed us photos that validated the intensity and speed of her physical decline.

Scientifically minded, Dr. Wahls decided to do her own research on her illness. She found that MS, Parkinson's, Huntington's, and Alzheimer's diseases all led to what she described as a "shrinking brain". She discovered a connection between the shrinking brain and the health of the myelin sheath. The myelin sheath is a protective coating around the neural fibers that send messages through our brains. This protective coating needs to be fully intact; when it is damaged, transmission of information within the brain cannot be completed.

This is a very complex system, but I have found a very simple way to help my students understand it on a very basic level. If you are interested, you can read more about it in the text box below, otherwise, feel free to skip the text box and move on.

Psychology 101 Refresher...

To explain the myelin sheath to my students, I use an analogy of insulation around water pipes during the most frigid and freezing winters. The insulation around the water pipes is like the protective coating around the neural fibers in our brains.

With this image in your mind, imagine that a rodent slowly rips away chunks of the insulation around your water pipe. In time, as the insulation is removed, the water in that section of the pipe will freeze. Once a section is frozen, water can no longer get from the tank to the faucets, tubs, or toilets. All transmission is stopped. This is similar to what happens in the brain when the myelin sheath is damaged.

The brain may try to send messages to move, react, or follow the topic of a conversation, but those messages never reach their final destination. When the protective coating of the myelin sheath is missing, the transmission is completely stopped.

In the reference list, you will find a link to Dr. Wahls web page and the video of the presentation that I saw in person.

The most fascinating key shared by Dr. Wahls is that we do not know enough about the micronutrients that our brains need to function at their best, nor do we know how various combinations of micronutrients interact to keep our brains healthy. Dr. Wahls personal search for a cure led her to adopt what she refers to as a "hunter-gatherer" diet. She reported positive changes within three months. Within nine months, she was riding a bicycle short distances. Eventually, she eliminated the need for a wheelchair, was walking without a cane or walker and said she was riding her bicycle to work again. Her truth was evident as she stood before us, showing photos chronicling the depths of her illness to her current recovery. She stood and moved across the stage in front of us without the aid of a cane, a walker, or a wheelchair.

As I listened to Dr. Wahls, there was one vegetable that she mentioned many times. This magic vegetable was KALE! She said it contained a multitude of necessary micronutrients that "feed mitochondria" which, in turn, support the protective coating around the neural fibers in our brains.

I knew I should not completely change my grandma's diet. Drastically changing a diet without the assistance of nutritional or dietary professionals can lead to any variety of digestive problems. It's also never a good idea to mess up a physiological system that is working well.

Luckily for me, my grandma's digestive system worked and ran like a Swiss watch - always perfectly on time. I did not want to change to a full "hunter-gatherer" diet overnight, but I could certainly add kale to our current diet. At best it might repair, slow, or minimize the damage that Alzheimer's was causing. At the worst, we would eat a vegetable that we never ate before and there would be no change at all. The advantages to be gained made eating kale a gamble worth taking.

I bought a bag of pre-washed kale and found a variety of ways to add it to every meal. At breakfast, I mixed it with scrambled eggs. At lunch, I put a cup-full into our soup. At dinner, I mixed it with rice. We each ate a cup of kale with every meal.

During this time, no other changes were made to Grandma's diet or routines. Within three weeks (coincidentally similar to the timeframe in which Dr. Wahls noted positive changes related to her illness) there was a notable improvement in my grandma's short-term memory.

Prior to this addition to her diet, Grandma was notorious for coming out of her bedroom with her slippers on the wrong feet. Every morning, with a few unconscious moans and groans, she shuffled slowly out of her room. Her eyes were usually half-opened as she methodically pushed her walker and made her way to the bathroom.

Every morning I would ask her, "Do your feet hurt?"

Her answer was short, "A little bit."

I'd say, "Look at your feet. Maybe they hurt because your shoes are on the wrong feet."

We would both laugh and I'd remind her to switch her shoes to the correct feet when she went to the bathroom.

This event happened almost daily for months on end. She never remembered to switch her shoes to the correct feet. She'd come out of the bathroom, shoes still on the wrong feet, and I'd say, "Hey, do your feet hurt?"

"A little." she'd say, as she made her way to the kitchen table.

As if for the first time, I'd say, "Maybe it would help if you put your shoes on the right feet."

She'd laugh and say, "Oh yeah. I think you told me that before."

With a silent sigh inside my mind, I thought, "Yes. I tell you that every day, twice a day." Of course, I would never say that out loud. Pointing out those details only reminds a loved one of their mental losses, and that leads to depression. Even if it's meant as a joke or said in a joking fashion, no matter how much you want to say those things, it's very important to keep them to yourself.

Besides the shoe problem, there was another common interaction that occurred during our breakfasts. My German shepherd loved to sit next to Grandma as she ate. At various points throughout breakfast, Grandma would sweetly reach out her hand and pet our beautiful 75-pound dog saying, "Good Kitty. You're such a good kitty."

For those of you who are full-time caregivers, you will realize that what I'm about to share is equally miraculous.

After three weeks of adding kale to every meal, my grandma came out of the bathroom with her shoes on the right feet and she began to consistently and correctly refer to the dogs as "doggies" and the cats as "kitties!" This was in no way a scientific study but I can assure you, it is true and her short-term memory improved. There was only one variable that changed, and that was the addition of kale to her daily diet.

It appears that Dr. Wahls was on the cutting edge of breakthroughs when she gave attention to diet as a means to keep our brains healthy. In the years since Dr. Wahls Ted talk, there have been additional studies that point to the power of nutrition on our brains and its connection to Alzheimer's and dementia. For example, new research points to evidence that our brains need insulin in order to fully function. Insulin resistance is now highly associated with an inability to think clearly. These studies are finding a strong connection between people with Type 2 diabetes and dementia. You can see some of the doctors, researchers, and patients involved with these studies in a 2013 Netflix documentary titled *"Untangling Alzheimer's."*

The bottom line is this: what we eat fuels our brains as much as gasoline fuels our cars. Think about what happens when dirt or other particles get mixed in with the gasoline in your car. Ask a mechanic what happens if sugar gets into the gasoline in your car (the simple answer = it kills it). Compare that to what we eat – (including the high levels of sugar in our daily diets) and the entire process is pretty easy to understand. Feed your brain, and your loved ones brain, with foods that are natural. Keep this simple rule in mind: the least processed it is, the better it is for you!

- *Kale- helpful hint 1: Baby kale is not bitter and can be eaten as a fresh salad. It can be used to replace lettuce on sandwiches or any other dishes that use fresh lettuce or spinach.*
- *Kale- helpful hint 2: Kale is like spinach. It gets stuck between your teeth. Make sure that you*

have toothpicks handy if you eat kale and plan to go out in public afterward.

- *Hint to keep up with Dr. Wahls advice and research: A link to her main webpage is located in the reference section of this book.*

Signs Minimize Confusion and Help Strengthen Neural Pathways

THERE IS A common cliché that parallels the current understanding of neural pathways in the brain; that cliché is 'Use it or lose it.' The more you use a specific pathway, the stronger it becomes.

Imagine that you are cutting a thick piece of wood with a steak knife. Every time you run the knife across the wood, the cut becomes deeper and more defined. This is similar to strengthening a neural pathway – making it stronger more defined. The more often you do something (for example - running the knife against the wood) the more defined and reinforced that pathway becomes. Based on the concept of brain plasticity, it's a logical conclusion that providing some basic information in a variety of places can help to build new neural pathways and improve short-term memory.

"Where's the bathroom?" or "Where's my room?" are questions you'll hear many times. Remember, this is a new home for your loved one. The answers to these questions are new information for him or her. However, for you, it's easy to become frustrated and angry after answering those questions over and over and over again. You might think, "Why are you trying to drive me crazy? I just told you that ten seconds ago." Instead, take a breath, stay calm, and remember that these questions are honest and sincere every time they are asked of you.

Trade places for a minute and try to think about what happens to the thoughts of our loved ones when we are not in the room. Imagine the feeling of confusion when they do not recognize anything at all. They often think, "This isn't my home." Next, they will begin to ask, "Who knows I'm here?"..."When can I go home?"

Waking up in a strange place with strange people could be a nightmare that leads to panic, frustration, and anger. Now imagine that nightmarish terror occurring multiple times a day. Any time there is no one in the room to answer your questions you feel anxious and fearful. Your mind races, trying to find answers, "Where am I?"..."How did I get here?"..."Is anyone coming to get me?"..."I just want to go home."

Keeping this in mind helps us to understand why many Alzheimer's and dementia patients become confused, angry, abusive, or depressed. The good news is that you can ease the confusion and anxiety as you help to build and strengthen the new neural pathways.

You can reduce the stress of this re-occurring nightmarish experience. You can help your loved one gain a sense of independence by creating informational systems so that he or she does not need you in the room in order to answer these questions.

Simple and easy-to-read directional and informational signs can provide answers every waking minute of every day! Every time these questions are asked, you simply point to a sign and ask, "What does that say?" In time (remember the knife cutting the wood), your loved one will begin to look for the signs instead of asking you for answers.

This process is powerful for a number of reasons:

- First, it encourages your loved one to read and think; keeping those neural pathways strong.
- Second, it alleviates momentary feelings of fear and confusion that come with being in a strange and foreign place.
- Third, it encourages a new learned behavior; looking for a sign to discover where the

bathrooms or bedrooms are located.

- Finally, it helps your loved one gain a sense of independence and control by not needing someone else to answer seemingly simple questions.

As an example, I had two signs in the kitchen that read, "Bessie's room." Each one had a photo of my grandma and a large black arrow that pointed in the direction of her room. She could see these signs easily, recognize herself in the photo, and follow the arrow to get to her room.

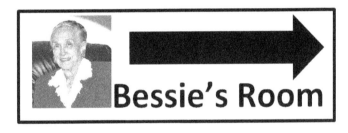

I had other informational signs in places that were always in my grandma's line of vision. For example, near my grandma's recliner chair, I had an 8 ½ x 11-inch sign. The first line read, "Bessie lives here with her firstborn granddaughter, Lisa." Next to this statement there was a photo of me and my grandma together so that she could recognize that we had a relationship. Seeing the photo with the easy-to-read text helped to remind her that this was "home." It helped remind her of who I was and it reminded her that she was in a safe place.

The second line read, "Friend Paula comes every day to have lunch and play games."

The last line read, "There is lots of love here." It was all very simple and direct information to help minimize the confusion that Alzheimer's brings.

Another sign was in the bathroom, in front of the toilet. This sign was in a lovely decorative frame that matched the colors and décor of the bathroom. Every time my grandma sat down on the toilet, she saw this sign. It had her favorite photo on it and it had only three statements:

- Bessie lives here, in Iowa, with her grand-daughter, Lisa.
- They have 3 dogs and 4 cats.
- This is a very happy home.

Even though my grandma had bounced around from family home to family home for a couple of years, these signs helped her to adjust very quickly. She knew this was her home now. Without first feeling lost or confused, she could get around the house to be in any room that she desired.

Feel free to use fancy framing that fits the décor of your rooms, but make sure the text (phrases or sentences) and lettering style (font) on your signs are visually simple.

Art and Design 101 Refresher...

Lettering styles are referred to as *fonts*.

Serifs are the little triangular edges seen on the letters of some fonts.

Some fonts have serifs and some do not.

"Sans" is a French word meaning without, thus, *sans serif* means without serifs.

Millions of people visit museums and most museums use fonts that are sans serif.

Take a closer look at most government-produced road signs. In the US, England, Canada, Mexico, Spain, and South Africa, road signs use fonts that are sans serif.

Serifs are lovely details but they can make reading a bit more difficult if vision is hindered by poor eyesight, poor lighting, or cloudy, foggy, or rainy days.

When I'm teaching art and design classes, I remind my students to consider the audience and the goal of the artwork or design.

When choosing between serif vs. sans serif fonts, consider this – How important is it for the reader to see, read, and comprehend your message quickly and accurately?

For our goal in making signs for our loved one:

- Use as few words as possible.
- Use black lettering on plain white, or off-white, paper.
- Use large, easy-to-read, sans serif fonts.
- Among the most popular and easy to read sans serif fonts are Calibri and Helvetica.

For my grandma's signs, I used **Calibri** font in sizes ranging from 36 to 72. You may be tempted to try some fancy lettering or typefaces such as *Brush Script* or Gothic, but studies show that these are more difficult to read. Think about road and highway signs. Lots of money goes into researching and choosing those simple typefaces with good reason: everyone needs to be able to read them quickly and accurately. We need to decipher the difference between an "I" and an "L" or a "T" and a "J". Don't give in to the temptation to show off how many fonts are on your computer. Keep it simple with large, bold, sans serif, black print on white or off-white paper.

I created my signs as 8.5 x 11 Microsoft Word documents and printed them on my simple home printer. Then I put them in frames that matched the décor in each room. Some signs were hung on walls, others were in self-standing frames, but they were all within Grandma's view from her favorite chair in each room.

- *Helpful hint #1: Use photos of your loved one that he or she likes of him or herself. My grandma loved the photo used here because her hair looked exactly as she liked it and she was wearing one of her favorite white lace blouses. She was dressed up and she liked to see herself that way. Using this photo made her want to look at these signs more often. I used this photo on many signs. Using the same (favorite) photo is also helpful – it's more quickly recognized by your loved one.*
- *Helpful hint #2: Test your signs before you buy frames and hang them up. Stand or sit where your loved one will be standing or sitting. Make sure your signs are easy to read from across the room.*
- *Helpful hint #3: Consider removing the glass from the frames. Removing the glass will reduce glare and also keep everyone safe if the frame accidentally falls to the ground.*

TIP **4**

Giving Choices Offers a Sense of Control that Results in Happiness

IT DOESN'T MATTER if you're 15, 35, or 55 years old. No one likes to be told what to do. Imagine what it feels like to have worked over 40 years, purchased your own home, bought your dream cars, paid your bills, raised your children, and lived a good life. Now imagine that all you've earned and worked for is either gone or controlled by someone else. You live in someone else's home. You can't get in your car and drive anytime you want. You can't go out to purchase your own food. You don't even choose what to wear anymore. You worked your whole life to be responsible and independent. Now, you look around and nothing is yours. Someone is telling you what you can and can't do every minute of the day. The person tell-ing you what to do may love and care for you – but that does not make it feel any better.

Try to imagine how powerless and depressing your waking hours might be. When Alzheimer's has led to full-time, in-home care, this is an example of how love is not enough to keep life happy for anyone. The loved one can become sad and depressed (with good rea-son) and that can lead the caregiver to feel unappreci-ated. A bad cycle of negative emotions has begun.

Numerous studies prove that everyone feels empow-ered and happier when they can make decisions for themselves.

When caring for an elderly loved one there is much to be accomplished: getting dressed, eating, maintaining personal hygiene, the list goes on and on.

Giving choices is a simple way to empower your loved one. Without question, this makes life easier and hap-pier for everyone.

A very simple key to letting your loved one feel em-powered is to offer two options for events that must be accomplished. To keep this simple, direct and easy, offer only two options (or choices). The answer to the option cannot be "Yes" or "No." here is the difference:

"Grandma, do you want to play a game?"

Her reply could be, "No. I'm tired." In this scenario, Grandma continues to watch TV, not exercising her brain or her body.

The difference in wording - to offer two options - goes like this:

"Grandma, do you want to go out for a walk **or** would you rather play a game of Scrabble?"

In this scenario, an activity (either *this* or *that*) is going to happen; "No" is not an option and no one is telling her "you need to do this." Grandma also understands that she gets to choose which of those options will happen. Grandma chooses and I follow her choice. By letting her choose the activity, she has a feeling of control over what is going to happen. With this sense of control, Grandma is happier and much more willing to complete the activity.

Here are some simple ideas to help provide choices, empowerment, and happiness in your home:

When getting your loved one dressed, put two outfits together and ask, "Which one of these outfits would you like to wear today?"

For some reason, Grandma began to hate taking a

shower. She especially hated washing her hair. When asked, "Do you want to take a shower now?" the answer was a definitive, "NO!" To address this problem, the following example worked for me:

I began to ask, "Would you like to take your shower now or in an hour from now?" and then she would make a choice.

Your loved one may forget the agreement, but at the agreed-upon time, you can remind him or her that (s) he made the choice and that might help. When short-term memory is nonexistent, it's helpful to have tangible validation of an agreement. There are a couple of things that you can do to help provide the validation needed.

One idea is to ask your loved one to write a note (or you write the note and ask for a signature). The note would simply say " I, __(signature of loved one)__ will take a shower at 11 a.m." At 10:30 a.m. you give a reminder, "Hey Grandma, it's 10:30 and you said you would take a shower at 11 a.m. okay?" At 10:45 give another reminder and at 11 a.m., show the signed note and hopefully, you will not have to argue about it.

Another idea, using current technologies on most cell phones, is to record a quick video of your loved one agreeing to whatever needs to be done and then playing it for your loved if he or she debates the issue.

These simple but powerful tools will help ease feelings of confusion and conspiracy. You can help to avoid these feelings by showing clear evidence of the agreement; helping to prove that you are not forcing something to happen just because you want it.

For meals, offer an option: "We have two vegetable choices for dinner – carrots or green beans - which one would you like?"

If your loved one is like my grandma, he or she will want to eat less "real food" and eat more ice cream and candy. Admittedly, in the beginning, I wasted a good amount of time arguing and debating with Grandma about her nutritional needs and the value of eating "real food" first, and ice cream second.

It was difficult for me to have these conversations because it made me feel like a hypocrite. Growing up, I was one of those kids who hated eating dinner. I still remember the hours of being forced to sit at the table to eat something that I didn't want to eat. I remember the lack of control in these situations. The reward of dessert, if I finished my dinner, was not enough to make me eat. Since I could not leave until I was done eating, I usually fell asleep at the dinner table. For me, dinner meant that the day was over and eating "real food" became a sad experience.

These memories led me to figure out a way to help

Grandma want to eat – rather than feeling forced to eat. I realized that the answer was in giving choices. With choices, arguing and debating is completely avoidable!

To help inspire my grandma to eat a healthy portion of "real food" before ice cream, I put the same amount of food on a dinner plate and also on a salad plate. Visually, on the smaller salad plate, the amount of food looked enormous. On the dinner plate, that same amount of food appeared to be much less.

I would show my grandma both plates of food and ask, "Which one of these would you like to eat?"

Believing that it was less food, she usually chose the dinner plate. Having this choice empowered her. Rather than feeling forced to eat a large portion of food, in her mind, she chose and received a "smaller portion" and she was happier. Daily life was easier, happier, and healthier when Grandma was empowered to choose which plate of food she wanted to eat. Feeling that she had control of what she ate gave her the perception of control. She was happier. Because she was happier, I was happier too.

In the area of health psychologically, there are many studies that prove it is **the perception of control** that is a big key to both health and happiness. It's a concept that is similar to the placebo effect.

Psychology 101 Refresher...

The easiest way to explain the power of the placebo effect is to think of reality in this way: "If you believe it's true, it is true." Placebos are used to test new drugs before they are available to the public. They are usually pills that look like the real drug, but the placebos do not have the active ingredient being tested. The people receiving the placebo believe that they are taking the real drug with the active ingredient.

Scientists use placebos to test if a drug actually works or if it is **the patient's belief** in the drug that makes it work. Quite often, people show improvement from taking placebos. This provides evidence that "if you believe something to be true, <u>it is true for you</u>."

Regarding a sense of control and empowerment in your daily life, **<u>your perception of control</u>** is all that matters.

One of the most powerful videos that I show in my psychology classes is a "Ted talk" by a Stanford researcher, Kelly McGonigal. The Ted talk is titled "*How to make stress your friend.*" This is a favorite for everyone because it brings many key concepts into clear focus. In everyday language, with easy to understand examples, this video explains the realities of how your thoughts and beliefs have a huge impact on your physical health and happiness. In the reference list, you will find a link to this Ted talk video that I show in my classes.

This research is related to concepts that might be referred to as locus of control, placebo effect, mindfulness, self-efficacy, or perception of control. The unifying factor among these concepts is the understanding that each person has the power to choose his or her beliefs and reactions to events in life.

For our purposes, remember that you are giving a sense of control in order to keep life manageable and happy. These changes in approach take only a few minutes but they can provide immeasurable happiness. In this way, you have the power to give your loved one, and yourself, a key to many more happy days!

Some people might see this as a deception. For example, putting the same amount of food on both plates might seem like a trick. Other people might feel bad for not being completely honest about the most current realities. If you are in this category, try to remember that the realities of someone suffering from Alzheimer's can be very different than your own. Your loved one does not have the same abilities to jump into current reality that he or she had before the illness began to take away connections to present-day existence. There are certainly moments of very clear and logical functioning, but those moments of clarity are fleeting. They may last a day, an hour, or only a few minutes. Those moments occur less and less often as time moves forward.

It is much more common that we get only tiny pieces of logic and reasoning from our loved one. For example, in our early debates about eating "real food" before ice cream, a piece of Grandma's reasoning was this: "Ice cream is food – we eat it – so it's food." I would then try to explain the nutritional difference between "real food" and dessert – I know – how silly was I? As you can imagine, at the end of those debates, we were both frustrated and unhappy.

It is very important to remember that the key to your own mental health is to do your best to build and create as many moments of happiness and joy as you can. What may seem like a trick is really the means of removing confusing or sad moments and replacing them with happy and empowering moments. When you get moments of clarity, they are the moments for you to remember – moments for you to cherish in the present.

Your sanity and mental health are extremely important. You cannot take care of anyone without those basic components being strong and resilient. There are more powerful lessons for happiness in using the concept of reciprocal causality!

Psychology 101 Refresher...

Reciprocal Causality: I help my students remember the power of this concept by first learning that *reciprocity* is just a fancy word for the idea of "give and take" or "exchange." Next, I ask my students to think of the word "cause" as one action leading to another action. When you break the words up into their individual pieces, you now understand that *reciprocal causality* is this: when we give and take, we cause something to happen.

In the case of Alzheimer's, when you give someone a choice, this leads to a feeling of empowerment and happiness for both parties. When your loved one with Alzheimer's is happy and calm, this provides you with happiness and calmness as well...it is an example of reciprocal causality. Give a sense of control and happiness to your loved one and gain a sense of control and happiness for yourself!

Take that Walker – It's Your New Purse (or Wallet)

LET'S FACE IT, no matter how much it's needed, almost no one willingly uses a walker. Doctors, specialists and other health care professionals can advise or require the use of a walker, but I have yet to see anyone willingly use it as directed. Many people consciously take the risk of falling and breaking a knee or hip before they will use a walker. These aren't even people with Alzheimer's or dementia – they are people with fully functioning brains. As caregivers, to help our loved ones, and ourselves, we must change our views on this fantastic life-saving apparatus.

I have friends who have fallen, were seriously hurt, and still refused to use a walker! One friend chooses to hobble around in pain, complaining about having to walk long distances from the parking lot to the store. He insists on only going to restaurants or public places that do not have stairs. Using a walker is medically advised and would alleviate a great deal of strain on his joints. Using a walker would allow him to move more, keep his circulation stronger, burn more calories, and be healthier than he is right now. Instead, he chooses to live in constant pain – moving as little as possible, moaning, groaning and risking a dangerous fall with every painful step. Refusing to use a walker is clearly making him more unhealthy.

Another friend chooses to use crutches instead of a walker. Seriously? Have you used crutches? They hurt your underarms and it's extremely easy to slip and fall while using them on uneven or slippery surfaces. They are not designed for people who are unstable or injured on both sides of their bodies.

For someone who is unstable and has painful joints, using crutches adds problems on top of problems. People who love you constantly fear a fall. That fear spreads through everyone in the room – even to strangers in a public place where crutches are much more difficult to maneuver. Crutches get caught on anything from another person, to doorframes, to the legs of tables and chairs.

Using crutches when you should use a walker endangers everyone around you. Falling with those long sticks in your hands turns you into Godzilla destroying Tokyo – you become a big crashing monster, taking down and smashing everything in your path. People who love you will try to catch you. It's highly likely that they will get caught in the gravity of the fall. Still, as insane and dangerous as it is – I've seen it and it is very scary. No one is relaxed.

Maybe using crutches is less emotionally traumatic. Maybe it's preferable to be viewed as someone who is injured from skiing or playing basketball rather than someone with painful joints. Obviously, it is best to use some form of assistance rather than none at all, but really...let's not be afraid of the walker! Let's not be afraid of stability. Don't let pride be your downfall (that is accidentally funny) – puns intended.

We must embrace the safety and strength of the walker and encourage its use in any way we can! Yes...it serves us best to change our view now. **Someday, it will be our turn to use the walker!**

I have already begun to design mine. It will be bright red with yellow and blue flames shooting and swirling up from the neon yellow tennis balls on the bottom!

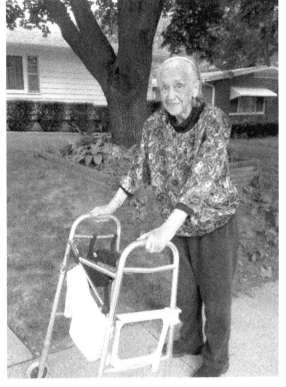

Photo credit: Linda Krug

I managed to get Grandma to use her walker by turning it into her purse! When the walker became her purse – holding all the things she liked to have handy – <u>she wanted to take it with her everywhere</u>.

In this photo, you can see one of my first attempts to accomplish this magical feat. I bought mesh pouches with zippers – the kind that are used to wash delicate clothing items in a washing machine. These can be found in the laundry aisles. I chose the mesh bags because I knew that I would not have to cut or poke holes into mesh bags – I could use the holes that already existed.

You can use clear plastic pouches if you like. Clear plastic pouches with zippers can be found in the aisles with suitcases and other travel items. I suggest using a corkscrew or paper hole puncher to make holes for the laces or zip ties that will hold the pouch securely to the walker. After you make the holes, you may want to put Super-Glue around the edges of the holes to strengthen them and minimize the opportunity for ripping to occur.

Whatever type of bag you choose, be sure to choose clear or mesh bags so that your loved one can visually see his or her items at all times. In the pouches, place items that your loved one needs or desires on a daily basis. This encourages your loved one to take the walker rather than leave it behind.

Sewing machines and messy glues are not needed for this project. Once you've purchased your pouches, use pipe cleaners, Velcro tape, zip ties, or long shoelaces to securely attach the pouches to the walker.

The choice of attachment-type will depend on what your loved one wants to put in those pouches. Heavier items will require more heavy-duty attachments. To add a touch of personality, choose these items in colors that your loved one wants to look at.

My grandma kept Kleenex, sugar-free hard candy, a protein bar, her eyeglasses, and at least five single dollar bills in her mesh bags. She was happy when she could see that she had her own money. If she was having a particularly good day, she would often offer me a dollar as a tip for my services.

She'd smile if I brought her coffee or a snack and say, "Oh, wait. I have something for you." Proudly unzipping her mesh bag, she would pull out a dollar bill and say, "Here honey. This is for you. You do such a good job taking care of me. I want you to have this."

At first, when this would happen, I would kindly decline, "Oh no. You keep that. I'm fine." But then I could see her pride quickly turn into sadness. I was not allowing her to express her strength or share her giving and thankful spirit. I was not allowing her to spend her money as she wanted. I was taking away her sense of control. I was not allowing her to feel empowered.

I learned to graciously accept the "tip", which I would sneak back into her bag when she took a nap.

- *Helpful hint #1: if you have pets in the house, be careful with the treat and food items that you put in these bags. Mesh bags might be too tempting for some furry family members. You might wake up to find that items are falling out of holes that were chewed in them as a furry family member decided to eat those tasty treats for a midnight snack!*

- *Helpful hint #2: buy reflective ribbon or tape and place this on the bag attachments or on the edges of the bags themselves. This will help your loved one see edges of the bags even if the light in the room is minimal.*

TIP **6**

Tame the Wild Raccoon Wandering Around the House at Night!

WHEN YOU'RE SLEEPING, an elder loved one with Alzheimer's can quickly turn into a wild raccoon wandering around, opening and getting into everything in your kitchen! One of the first "wild raccoon" events happened to coincide with my birthday.

A key piece of the story begins with me on the hunt for just one gift to myself that I could not find online. I wanted an "old-school Janet Jackson style" military jacket. Miraculously, on the day before my birthday, I found one of these jackets in my favorite heather grey color! It seemed that it was going to be a lovely birthday.

Rather than buy a birthday cake that I'd have to hide from my grandma (she was diabetic and I can't eat food with sugar substitutes), I had recently become addicted to Arby's Hershey's chocolate turnovers and that's all I wanted. I stopped at an Arby's and ordered two turnovers which would serve as my birthday breakfast the next day. The turnovers were right out of the oven - fresh, warm, and fluffy. The aroma filled the car as I drove home. I could already taste them! But I was going to postpone my enjoyment until the official morning of my birthday. I've been told that I "live in the moment" too much. I was going to prove to myself, and have evidence, that I could enforce a "grown-up" level of self-control.

As I put the bag of chocolate heaven in the cabinet above the microwave, I envisioned a perfectly peaceful birthday morning - waking up early and going downstairs to make my coffee. Grandma's favorite cat, Boombie, would be curled up in his wicker basket in the sun zone, waiting for Grandma to wake up so he could take his royal spot on her lap. As the sun poured in, beams of light would jump through the giant stained glass window and bounce off hanging crystals, sending rainbows of color in every direction.

Meanwhile, Grandma would be in her own private dreamland, snoring soundly. As I listened to those soft and even breaths, knowing Grandma was perfectly relaxed, I could relax too. With all of that in place, I could slowly savor my chocolate-filled dream breakfast. A perfect morning for a perfect day.

Afternoon birthday plans involved lunch with girlfriends and me in my new military jacket. I hung my new jacket on the back of a kitchen chair in order to keep it handy for the lunch outing. It was the perfect color, perfect size, and had perfect buttons - I smiled just looking at it – what a lucky find!

Before I went to bed that night, I triple-checked everything: nice clean kitchen, dishes washed and put away, nothing on the counters, chocolate heaven hiding in the cabinet, military jacket ready for my lunch outing - everything was perfectly in place for a cozy, calm, and delicious morning.

Psychology 101 Refresher...

To help explain the confusion of the actual birthday morning events, it's much more amusing if you first have a quick lesson in the psychology of personality according to Sigmund Freud:

Sigmund Freud is famous for many of his theories. Among them is his three-pronged

---

theory of personality. The essence of his theory claims that we have an ID, an ego, and a superego and this is how I explain it – in its most simple terms - to my students…

- The ID is a big spoiled selfish baby who wants what it wants and it wants it now.

- The superego is the opposite of the ID. It is the part of the personality that holds on to the guidelines for behavior that our parents and our society give us: the superego is what gives us the rules regarding the "right and wrong" of behavior.

- We also have the ego. This is not the same ego that we think of when we say, "He has a big ego." According to Freud, the ego is the part of the personality that tries to find a balance between the ID's selfish wants and society's rules that are held tightly in our superegos.

When you see this theory represented in cartoons, you'll recognize the ID as the devil on the shoulder, trying to get the human to do something that is completely self-serving. Regardless of all else, the ID screams ME, ME, ME. IT'S ALL ABOUT ME!

The angel, on the opposite shoulder, represents the superego. The superego is telling us to follow the rules and "do the right thing."

The ego has to find a way to balance the desires of the devil and the angel so that we can live our lives productively and feel good about what we have done.

As I tried to sleep that night, these three parts of my personality were having a ferocious battle. My ID kept trying to tear down my willpower. Over and over again it told me to "Eat a turnover now. Go ahead. Eat one. Just one. No one will know. You earned it." My ID was super sneaky, trying to justify the action by saying, "It's okay. You have two. You can still have one on your birthday." all the while knowing that if I ate one, I would eat them both! That ID can be quite a devilish little trouble maker!

My superego screamed in my head, "NO! The rules say that you have to wait until your real birthday! If you eat them now, you will feel guilty and you will not enjoy them. You'll feel terrible all night and you'll feel bad on your birthday."

My ego was in the middle, whispering the answer to

getting both. "You can do it. You can wait until tomorrow and it will feel better than eating them now. It's only a few hours away. You'll go to sleep and then wake up. It's not difficult. You can wait." I listened to my ego and chose to wait.

I woke up with the energy of a six-year old child and flew down the stairs so the birthday extravaganza could begin. Racing into the kitchen I was confused and dumbfounded when I encountered crumbs on the counter. The kitchen was spotless when I went to bed. For a fraction of a second, I wondered, "Where did this come from?"

My ID quickly took over, "Who freakin' cares? Eat a chocolate turnover right NOW!" In that moment, my ID won. I didn't care about anything else. I waited long enough and I had to have one of those delicious treats. As if I hadn't eaten in months, I flung open the cabinet door and grabbed the bag of turnovers.

"WHAAAAAAT the ????" The bag was EMPTY!

My mind raced, "Did we have mice? Did the dogs get in here? Where are my turnovers?"

Like a heat-seeking missile searching for a target, my eyes darted around the kitchen searching for answers to this hideous crime. As my heart rate slowed and sanity began to kick in, I began to see some clues:

1. The crumbs on the counter were definitely fluffy turnover crumbs!
2. Dark smudges of chocolate created a messy trail across the counter that was easy to follow.
3. The trail moved down to a dish-drying towel that was hanging on the oven door, and then I saw it. My heart stopped as my brain put the pieces together. I had to purposefully take a breath or I'd pass out as my head was spinning.
4. "NOOOOO!!!! No. No. No." It hurt to look at it. My new heather-grey military jacket had been used as a towel to wipe messy chocolate off the hands of a giant and naughty diabetic raccoon who wandered around, loose in the kitchen at night!

Shock quickly turned to fear as I ran into the bedroom to see if my grandma was in a diabetic coma. I shook her shoulder. "Grandma, Grandma, wake up! Wake up!"

It appeared that she used warm melted chocolate for warrior paint on herself and her bedding! Dark chocolate was streaked across her face, hands, pillow, sheets, and bedspread.

She wasn't moving. I shook her again. "Grandma, Grandma, wake up!"

She moaned. Her eyes tried to open. Thank goodness

she wasn't in a coma! Now I could allow myself to be angry.

"You ate my chocolate turnovers!" I screamed.

With absolute conviction that she was telling the truth, she said, "No, I didn't."

"Yes, you did! What's this all over your face and hands?" I tried to place one of her hands where she could see it. She was okay, but still too groggy to fully focus and open her eyes.

After a few minutes of insanity, I realized that my yelling was not helping anyone. She had absolutely no idea what was going on. Grandma, full of sweetness, was tired from her midnight snacking adventure. This beautiful raccoon found herself a chocolate jackpot in those turnovers – real chocolate – and that's something that she hadn't had in years!

I wiped the war paint off of her hands and face and left her sleeping soundly as I moved on to clean the kitchen. As the sun poured in and illuminated the destruction of my fantasy, I sat in a chair and cried. Two chocolate turnovers and a jacket were all I wanted. That seemed reasonable enough - it's not like I was asking for a new car or a trip to Bali. As a caregiver, your focus is on your loved one at all times. You care for them when they are awake and you worry when they are asleep. You do not make plans for yourself without considering your loved one. Will he or she be able to be alone for a few hours? Can you bring your loved one with you? Can you find reliable and trustworthy help? Your life has many moments when responsibility for your loved one supersedes your own wants.

I wasn't crying because of a silly jacket or a chocolate dessert for breakfast. I cried because I just wanted a few minutes for myself on a day when most people get a little bit of something special. I worked and planned for this particular morning to be perfect and, with all that planning, not one piece worked. I remember sitting down and feeling completely drained. It was as if I had just been unplugged from my power source.

I wanted to give up. I could not give up. Instead, I sat down and cried and that helped. It always helps - although I advise crying in the shower so you can be alone as long as needed and blow your nose without wasting a box of Kleenex! (If you feel like this – Please jump to the Bonus Tip at the end of this book and read that now!)

At that time in life, I told my friends that this birthday was ruined by 'Bessie the Raccoon' who was foraging through the kitchen at night. Today, I wish I could live that birthday a hundred times over. I would laugh to see so much chocolate all over the kitchen again and smile at how Grandma managed to get it all over her beautiful face. What once seemed like a disaster is now one of my most cherished memories!

Of course, Grandma should not have eaten all of the sugar at once. This "raccoon event" made me realize that she could have eaten anything and ended up in a diabetic coma. What if she ate a bunch of desserts that didn't leave clues for me to find? Not all sugary desserts will leave such easy to follow trails! This realization inspired an easy fix to help tame a wild raccoon at night.

After some trial and error, the quick and inexpensive solution that I voted for was to use clear packaging tape to keep the cabinet and refrigerator doors from being opened.

If you choose this solution, fold one edge so you have a "pull-tab" for yourself. Place the tape in a different location from the cabinet and refrigerator door handles.

You might think that the pull-tab would be easy for the beloved raccoons to figure out, but my grandma never did. She would pull on the handles and when the doors would not open, she would move on to another cabinet.

If the tape doesn't work, you can resort to childproof

cabinet locks. Personally, the installation and use of those quickly annoyed me. They pinched my hands and fingers and added frustration to days that didn't need any more of that.

I hope this quick and easy fix works for you too. Happy Birthday!

Ease versus Strength - Think Before You Choose

THERE ARE MANY technologies to make life easier by minimizing physical effort. With new technologies such as "Alexa" and "Echo Dots", many people no longer have to get out of a chair in order to manually turn off lights, radios, or lock doors. A simple verbal request such as, "Alexa, turn off the lights." will make it so. Other technologies, such as auto-lift chairs easily move a person from a seated to a standing position in seconds.

After Grandma had lived with me for a couple of months, with love and concern for her comfort, my Aunt Betty Anne brought a recliner chair for Grandma to use. Grandma loved it and I immediately moved things around to make it fit in our living room.

As soon as I saw it, it reminded me of episodes of the TV sitcom, "*Frasier*." If you've ever seen this long-running TV sitcom, you might remember the many debates and arguments that stemmed from the old recliner chair that Frasier's father, Marty, insisted on keeping. Frasier hated that chair, pointing out that it was covered with "duct tape and dog hair." Frasier attempted, many times, to remove or replace it simply because it did not match his very expensive decor. In the reference section, you will find a link to a clip of this episode which gives focus to the value of this chair. The scene is extremely powerful in helping caregivers understand things that our elderly loved might feel but never say.

This gift from my aunt immediately reminded me of Marty's chair – minus the duct tape. It didn't match anything in my home. This chair was all manual. There was no handle or electrical controls to make the footrest pop up. Grandma had to hold the armrests and push her body-weight back in order for the chair to recline. The chair had three positions: the fully seated chair position, the intermediate reclining position with footrest, and a fully reclined position that often led to a wonderful nap at any point in time.

In the beginning, Grandma maneuvered this chair with ease but with each passing year, it was clear to see that it took more and more effort for her to get this chair into a reclining position. Sometimes, it took Grandma three or four tries to fully recline with her feet up. Eventually, she had to stop and rest in between her attempts to recline. She was so tired and watching this became unbearable.

I began searching for an electric auto-lift recliner that would effortlessly move her from a standing to a reclining position, and back up again, with the simple push of a button. I searched for the perfect color, fabric, and ease of use for a variety of fully automatic recliner chairs but I kept going back to compare them to the manual recliner chairs. As I went back and forth, I began to realize the physical strength that was needed to maneuver the manual chair.

With some background and training in athletics, dance, and fitness, I had to face a complicated reality. If I bought my grandma an automatic recliner, she would no longer need to use her muscles and strength. Every day, getting in and out of her chair to use the restroom or go into the kitchen, required her to use her muscles. By eliminating this daily use of those muscles, in a very short time, she would become weaker.

In the later stages of Alzheimer's, other than walks up and down our block, the physical requirements of getting in and out of her chair became a major part of her daily movement routine. She needed this to stay strong.

It was still very difficult to watch her struggle to re-cline in her chair - taking breaks to rest before she tried again to push her body weight back in order to recline. Every now and then, she was out of breath enough that she would want to give up. "I'll just sleep sitting up." she'd say.

At these moments, I took on the role of Grandma's biggest cheerleader. "Come on Grandma. Don't give up. You can do it."

"Ughhh," she'd sigh, "I'm so tired. I can't do it. I'll just sit like this. I'm fine." By this point, her head and torso were usually leaning sideways. The armrests were the only things keeping her from falling or rolling out of the chair. She needed a cheerleader to bring back the fighting spirit of "Rosie the Riveter."

I'd remind her that she could do anything, "You can do it. I know you can. You're the strongest person I know." This always made her laugh. These pieces of positivity and humor are extremely important. Remember the concept of reciprocal causality (noted in Tip #4), if you sound positive and hopeful, that feeling can be shared and it can spread. It is much more helpful than a sad or negative tone.

With understanding, remembering times when I was the one exhausted beyond imagination, I'd say, "Okay, rest for a second and then give it one more big try. Give it all you've got. I know you can do it!"

After a few minutes, I'd ask, "Are you ready?!"

She was as enthusiastic as a child being told to eat mushy vegetables. After a long sigh, she would say, "Okay."

I'd say, "I'll count to three and then you push back really hard. Okay?"

To gain a few more seconds of rest, she'd slowly repeat the plan, "Okay…You count…And then I'll push."

As her cheer captain I'd shout, "One, two, three, PUSH!" and she was able to do it! The entire process of trials took about half an hour but in the end she was smiling, proud, exhausted, fully reclined, and ready for a well-earned nap.

This may sound like I tortured her, especially since there is so much assistive technology to alleviate the strain of these physical tasks. As tempting as it was, I never gave in to the lure of the automatic chair. I knew it would lead to a quick spiral of her becoming weaker instead of keeping the strength she had.

Instead of an automatic chair, I made some modifications to help her get in and out of her manual chair with greater ease. The first modification was to raise her seated position so that the movements in and out of the chair minimized the strain on her back and knees. I did this by putting additional cushions on her chair.

Through extensive trial and error, my advice is to use the semi-firm, plastic covered, memory foam type stadium seat cushions. These are the best for a number of reasons. First, they are firm enough to provide the added height needed (the body sinks into softer pillows and that only magnifies the problem). Second, they are "water/weather-proof". This is great when the reality of life is that most people in this age range "leak".

It is a sad truth that you will have to wash many loads of urine-soaked clothing, sheets, and blankets. Using these "water/weather-proof" seat cushions eliminates the need to constantly replace soft pillow-like seat cushions.

To add layers of protection and softness, I bought inexpensive vinyl tablecloths with felt backing. I put one of those over the cushions and then placed a towel on top of that. "Leaking" and its accompanying odor were no longer problems because accidents were easy to clean. All I had to do was wipe the vinyl tablecloth and plastic seat cushion with a disinfecting cleanser and replace the towel with a clean one.

In the end, Grandma had the perfect chair. She could sit down and get up on her own. Using her muscles enabled her to stay stronger longer.

For me - clean-up from any spills or accidents involving bodily fluids was quick and easy.

"Secret" Exercise Plans that Improve Physical Strength and Self-esteem

FOR MANY PEOPLE in their 80s and 90s, simply getting up to use the restroom seems like a grueling work-out. It's imperative to keep the blood flowing throughout the brain and body. In the aging process, it's natural that everything slows down.

These next tips have a two-fold purpose. First, they get your loved one moving and get the blood flowing for an extended period of time. Second, they give your loved one a sense of purpose: a feeling of being a contributing member of the household rather than a burden to you. All of this leads to feelings of self-worth and happiness.

The easiest way to encourage "secret exercising" is to let your loved one fold towels. I was working in the adult psychiatric unit when I first came up with this plan. We had an elderly patient who was depressed and not very mobile. During a particularly busy shift, I walked by her many times as she sat in her wheelchair in the hallway – just sitting there, looking sad. I must have looked tired because eventually, she asked if she could help me. She was bored. Her tone and facial expression told me that she needed something to do.

It was a busy shift. I couldn't play a card game or sit and talk, but I wanted her to feel good, happy, and valuable. I ran to the linen closet, grabbed an armful of washcloths and piled them on the table beside her. I said, "It would be a great help if you could fold these for me." Her eyes lit up and she began folding. She used a variety of motor skills as she picked up each towel, shook it out, folded it, and placed one on top of the others to build a neat and balanced stack.

I continued to give her this job every day. With every towel-folding assignment she was smiling and her mood improved almost immediately. She had a job. She had value. She felt needed and she was in control of working as fast or as slow as she wanted. Remember a key point from Tip #4 - perception of control is a huge key to happiness!

For my grandma, I'd provide a variety of towel sizes:

washcloths, dish towels, bath sheets and everything in between. This necessitated a variety of arm movements and cognitive functions as she worked to place similar sized towels in their own piles. She loved this "job." In an instant, rather than feeling like a burden, she became a contributing member of the household.

My grandma also loved to wash the dishes. I admit that this was a difficult job to allow at first. I was concerned that she would drop something and hurt herself. I became increasingly concerned when I watched her wash dishes without using any soap or cleanser. At first I monitored her every move, verbally reminding her to use soap or rinse an item again. This process left both of us feeling frustrated.

The "happy ending" came when I realized the goal was <u>not</u> to end with clean dishes! The goals were to get my grandma moving and to help her feel valuable. I stopped watching her and I stopped giving her directions. My new reality was that Grandma helped by pre-washing the dishes after every meal. She was a contributing member of our home.

When Grandma would wash the dishes, I would leave the kitchen in order to encourage her sense of independence. When I left the kitchen, I would make an announcement such as, "I'll wait for you in the living room and we'll watch whatever you want when you're done." She liked knowing that I trusted her and that she did not need a babysitter. She did not feel like a burden. She was contributing, working, and helping and that made her very happy.

Later in the day, when she took her naps, I re-washed the dishes, but she didn't need to know that part. Getting her moving and feeling productive was all that mattered.

Another easy exercise plan is to encourage your loved one to brush the hair of any pets in your home. Hand muscles are used while holding the brush and a variety of muscles in the arm are used in the long sweeping motions. Depending on the size of your pet, the brushing movement can activate many muscle groups in the fingers, hands, arms, and shoulders.

All of our pets loved to be brushed. This was a win-win for everyone: Grandma got some exercise and pets got attention. There was the added bonus of a calm and peaceful aura that was created with Grandma feeling needed and valued. Like the dishes, this was another important "job" that needed to be done on a regular basis. Being able to do it without receiving verbal directions gave her a sense of independence, and that added to her happiness as well.

In the photo below, you can see Grandma with Frankie. Frankie LOVED to be petted by Grandma. In this photo, you can see what I saw every day in my living room. Frankie, while lying on her own couch, would get as close to Grandma as possible. Then, Frankie would roll upside down and begin to whine for attention. Sometimes, Grandma tried to ignore Frankie, but this was impossible. Frankie can cry and whine for over an hour! Grandma always gave in. You can see in this photo how Grandma had to stretch in order to reach over the armrests and pet Frankie. You can see also see Grandma's big smile in being able to make Frankie happy.

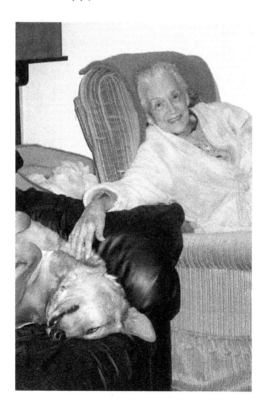

This was another easy way for Grandma to get some exercise. The stretching and reaching toward Frankie helped to increase Grandma's range of motion and it never felt like work or exercise to her. She loved to spoil all the pets in our house - which leads to another hilarious story with lessons that you'll get to read in Volume II. For now, we'll move on to Tip # 9 and the incredible power that music can have on our memories.

Use Music as a Memory Enhancer!

MUSIC AND ITS associated emotional memories are stored through a vast array of networks in the brain. Because of this, music has a magical ability to bring about powerful feelings and clear memories from years gone by. It may seem like science fiction, but there is ample observable data to support the powerful influence that music can have on both emotions and memories.

Think about music in your own life. There are certain songs that take you right back to high school. Songs that take you back to that first kiss or that first car. Maybe there are songs that remind you of a particular vacation. I know that any time I hear reggae music,

I'm right back in Jamaica – walking on the beach, drinking a frozen chocolate mudslide!

Music has power. Some songs make us happy. They can make us move without thinking. Even people who don't want to dance can't help tapping a finger on a table, or a foot on the floor, when they hear a favorite song or rhythm.

The power of music to "awaken sleeping areas of the brain" is wonderfully expressed in a 2014 documentary titled *Alive Inside: A Story of Music & Memory*. You can easily obtain this documentary from any public library. If it's not in stock, you can request that it be sent to your library through inter-library loan (a free service). There is more than enough evidence to show that reviving memories and bringing back happy times, especially for loved ones suffering from Alzheimer's, may be as easy as playing music from cherished decades.

Even in popular culture, there is a wonderful tribute to the power of music on memory. I recently watched Disney/Pixar's award-winning animated film "*Coco*". In this film, Coco is the great-grandmother with Alzheimer's disease. The theme of the film is focused on understanding the Day of the Dead and showing how this celebration honors our ancestors. It's a lovely way to help deal with the loss of our loved ones. As an added bonus, in this film, the power of music on memory is made clear.

Near the end of this film, there is a powerful scene where the grandson sings to his great-grandma. When he begins, her eyes are closed and her head is hanging down. The song he sings has emotional power and is connected to vivid memories from her childhood. As Great-Grandma Coco hears the melody, she begins to brighten up in every way. She picks her head up and begins to open her eyes. She smiles. Great-Grandma Coco begins to sing the song too and is then able to recall more and more details of the father who loved her.

It's true that this is fictional animation, but it is a clear representation of something that we DO know for sure – that music has a powerful and direct connection to distant memories. When you understand this, and you are caring for a loved one suffering from memory deficiencies, you can use this knowledge to create many more happy moments in your days!

The key to remember is that the music played must be of <u>emotional value to your loved one</u>. You may not know this detail but it's fairly easy to figure out. Ask your loved one to tell you about some of his or her favorite times of life. Was it free and easy childhood or teen years? Was it the years of having a young family? Ask! If you don't get a clear answer, ask again later. Ask again on another day. Remember that those moments of clarity will come and go. Don't give up.

If verbal responses are not at their highest, try using visual cues. Show photos of special moments. Show photos of places your loved one may have visited on a special vacation. Figure out the year that special moment took place. Use that place and timeframe as the basis of your search to find the memory-enhancing music that is perfect for your loved one.

Once you have a time frame, do a quick online search for the *Top 40 Musical Hits* of that year or decade. Play a few songs. See what happens. Keep experimenting until you find what works best to bring about happy thoughts and memories. Seeing fingers tapping on a table is a good sign that you're on the right track. Who knows, you may even see some fancy dance moves!

In regard to my grandma's favorite music, I knew that she loved to dance the polka and that she used to drive as far as Nebraska in order to go to Czech polka festivals. Since I don't speak the Czech language and I know absolutely nothing about polka music, I had to buy a few CDs and test them with her. I played Czech polka music every day at breakfast and lunch. No matter what her feelings were when she sat down, the music usually inspired her to smile and tap her feet. We listened to a few CDs, but there was one that always took her back to her childhood when she spent very happy summers with her own grandma. She would hear the songs, sing-along, and then ask, "Can you take me to see my grandma today?"

Some health-care professionals still insist on correcting the patient/client to be in the current real moment and time of life. I refer to this as the *"reality policy."* In this example, with my grandma wanting to visit her grandma, the directive of the reality policy would be to bring Grandma into our reality. The reality policy dictates that I kindly inform my grandma of her age and that her own grandmother is no longer alive – bring Grandma into the current time and reality of life right now.

I absolutely disagree with this approach. In real life, this approach adds additional trauma and frustration to days where patience and understanding may already be strained to the breaking point for everyone. Sadly, I have seen and heard of many instances where the directive to "correct" the Alzheimer's client was strictly enforced.

A real-life example involves a caregiver at the senior-care facility where I took my grandma on days when I had to work late. One day, my grandma and another woman (we'll call her "Trudy") were the last two clients at the center. Trudy was waiting near the front door, looking out of the windows, and asked the caregiver, "What time will my husband be here to get me?" The caregiver knew Trudy's husband was dead and that her son that was coming to get her. Rather than cause emotional trauma with the *reality policy*, the caregiver told Trudy that her son was coming to pick her up because her husband was out of town. Trudy easily accepted this explanation and remained calm as she continued to stare out the window, waiting for her son.

According to senior daycare policy, the caregiver should have corrected Trudy's beliefs by telling her that her husband was no longer alive. Following policy, the caregiver should have reminded Trudy that she was a widow who now lived with her son. The caregiver was verbally reprimanded and formally written-up for not following the "reality policy".

Why did the reality policy need to be enforced here? How is life better if Trudy is reminded that her husband is dead? Her son was on his way to pick her up. After a long day at work, does it help the son to remember his own father's death? It forces him to re-live it as much as it forces his mom to believe it. What additional stress and trauma would Trudy's son have to deal with if he is rewarded with the joy of driving home, explaining to his mother, again, that her husband was dead and that she no longer had her own home? What good comes from reminding Trudy of these sad truths? Imagine the confusion, anger, and sadness that accompany these realities.

Do these realities make life better? Do they make an Alzheimer's patient safer or happier? Do such truths and realities lead to understanding or trust? Do they add anything positive or beneficial to the quality of life? Is anyone honestly helped or made better by using this approach?

In the case of my grandma wanting to see her own grandma, I would simply ask more questions and begin to change the focus. I would ask, "Where does your grandma live?", "What does her house look like?", "Are there animals there?", etc. Instead of a focus on going to visit my great-grandma, the focus moved on to discussing happy memories of the summers that my grandma spent with her grandma.

If my grandma remained insistent on a visit to her grandma, I would say that her grandma was visiting family in the Czech Republic right now. Because this side of my family immigrated from Czechoslovakia, this thought was absolutely plausible and it made my grandma very happy.

These moments of memory loss become more frequent. The same question might be asked ten times in a row, over and over and over again. Every time you give the answer, you are choosing the emotional outcome for everyone in your home. Remember the theories of reciprocal causality and the power of choice noted in Tip #4? Here are those same theories in action again. What answer inspires peaceful feelings? Will the realities of accurate time and place bring smiles, or will they lead to sadness and frustration?

It's true that my system may be in opposition to policies at some elder-care facilities, but when you put the emotional realities of your everyday real-life up against this *"reality policy"*, I'm here to remind you that, in your home, YOU get to choose.

As yet, I have not read research that shows cognitive or emotional improvements when using this type of reality approach. Will you choose to live in moments of peace and calm or will you choose to constantly correct your loved one – bringing him or her to the current realities of life today? This decision is yours and yours alone. This tip for living more calmly on a day-to-day basis has a direct connection to Tip #10.

Enter the Worm-hole to Another Dimension and Allow Life to be Exciting!

THIS TIP IS an extension of Tip #9. This tip encourages something that does more than eliminating or minimizing sad moments – it actually creates exciting ones! And better yet, it's absolutely FREE!

Take a moment to pause and look around at your current environment. Think about your routines. Think about someone you see on a daily basis: a spouse, child, or neighbor. Imagine that you expect to see that person in the next few minutes but someone tells you that person has been dead for years. How would that make you feel? Would you believe that person? Would you question his or her sanity?

Quite often, Alzheimer's victims are corrected in their assessments of time and place. They are told that they are wrong about the decade, year, and other current events that are at the forefront of their minds. With these constant corrections, it's common for them to feel confused.

Try to trade places for a minute. If this happened to you – someone telling you that your belief about where you are, what year it is, or who you're with, is wrong. You might think it's a conspiracy to drive you insane. You might begin to distrust the very person who is caring for you and loves you dearly. You can't help but feel distrustful when you think you know where you are but this "stranger" is telling you that you're wrong. You think you know who is dead and who is alive, but your mind has played a hiding game with big chunks of your memories. Little by little, as the "stranger" provides more and more proof of the current realities - showing you photos or newspapers, pulling up a page on the internet, or turning on a current TV news station - you might begin to question yourself. In a flash, everything you believed to be true has been proven wrong. There are decades that you don't remember. People you loved are gone. With this dose of current reality, you are likely to feel confused, frustrated, depressed, or angry.

Now, imagine that these moments of reality are being

forced upon you all the time! How do you feel about life now? Are you happy? Is it easy to just accept these realities and move on to have a happy day?

Even though I rarely corrected my grandma to current time and place, there were times when I corrected her without thinking about it. After I made the corrections, I could see the sadness take over as she realized that her memory was slipping. These moments bothered me greatly. I thought about them often – trying to figure out how I could minimize them. Finally, as if an outer force downloaded a giant instruction manual into my brain, I had a flash of inspiration. This was a powerful turning point and it began with a series of very similar days.

This series of similar days began when I was giving presentations to large groups of professional educators all week long. For my presentations, I was wearing my best designer suits to work every day. When I came home, my grandma saw me walk through the door in high heels and a fabulous suit that was rarely seen. You know the ones – those special suits stored in their own special clothing bags – waiting for a special event – I was wearing those suits all week.

When she saw me walk through the doorway, she would light up. With a big smile, she'd ask, "How was New York?"

Of course, I had no idea what she was talking about so the automatic response was, "I didn't go to New York. I'm just coming home from work."

"But you're in a fancy suit and shoes? I thought you were in New York. Didn't you just come home from New York?"

Again, without thinking, I replied, "Nope - just had to give a presentation today. I've been in Iowa all day long."

The gleam in her eyes quickly dwindled as she quietly said, "Oh." and looked away.

This happened for three days in a row.

As I drove home on the fourth day, I thought about these interactions. I hated seeing my grandma get sad when she realized I had not gone to New York. It made me sad that these corrections made her realize that her mind was slipping away. I drove past miles of cornfields on the way home but her sad face was all I could see. I didn't want to see it another day.

I thought, "She's going to ask me about New York. Why can't I be coming home from New York? That's much more exciting than coming home from a presentation in Iowa!"

With this revelation, life took a drastic change for the better. I was anxious to get home. I ran up the steps to get inside to see her and see if life could be happier, starting tonight.

As expected, as soon as she saw me, she perked up and asked, "How was New York?" I gladly stepped into the worm-hole and entered her reality. With big eyes and a huge smile, I was almost out of breath as I said, "It was fabulous! I went to a Broadway show and bought some amazing shoes that they don't have here in Iowa!"

My grandma was a fashion statement in her day. She loved seeing live shows and she loved shoes. I knew both of these details would be exciting for her. She honestly wanted to hear more about them.

For the next twenty minutes or so, we would talk about all the fun things to do in New York. Luckily, I had been there so I was able to share true events. It was great fun to listen to her stories and to see her smiling and happy as she recalled details of her travels. During these times, we shared many adventures. Rather than forcing my grandma into the realities of my current life (simply giving presentations in Iowa all week long), I allowed myself to enter the current experience in her mind.

I allowed myself to let go of the constraints of my real

life and walk through the Alzheimer's worm-hole to join her in her experience. Truthfully, joining her was so much more fun! As a bonus, I was able to learn more about her travels - things I had not known before.

From that day forward, whenever I walked through the door in a fancy suit, we shared stories about New York. Every day after that, fancy suit or not, I did my best to join my grandma's current reality rather than force her into mine.

In your daily life, as you care for this person you love, ask yourself these questions: Why is it that only children or science fiction writers are encouraged to imagine new realities? Will life stop or will someone be endangered if you allow it to be 1953, or if you're in a cruise ship cabin instead of a tiny bedroom? Wouldn't life be happier if a long-departed spouse, friend, or relative is believed to be alive on a business trip or on a vacation instead of dead? Must you have a debate or argument over such things? Will it improve the quality of life?

If the belief does not endanger your loved one, take a little jump into the Alzheimer's worm-hole. You might find that life is a bit more exciting there!

BONUS TIP: Don't try to go it alone!

NO MATTER HOW much love you have to give, you need time away to rejuvenate. You MUST take some time to care for yourself. It doesn't need to be a full week on an island (although that would be nice) - it only needs to be a few hours away from the house: a short break once a week is a good goal. When you can get away for 2 or 3 hours, knowing that your loved one is safe, your mind and body can truly relax and re-energize!

Honestly, after months of "smooth" caregiving 24/7, it is highly likely that you will not realize how much you need a break, but once you have even two hours of mental and emotional rest, you will feel the difference. You will be "the best you" instead of the "just functioning" you.

I was very lucky to have my Aunt Marianne help in this regard. The first time she suggested coming to Iowa to take grandma away for the weekend and give me a break I thought, "That's crazy. Why would you want to do that? She's fine. We're fine and I don't need a break." Grandma and I had found our rhythm in life and I was afraid to mess that up. Luckily, my aunt insisted on having it her way.

Even though she works many hours and lives four hours away, she and one of her best friends, Michael, would drive to Iowa to whisk Grandma away for entire weekends at a time. Grandma got a mini-vacation to a favorite nearby casino and she always got to see live dancing - Marianne and Michael are swing dance experts. Wherever they went, they managed to find a dance floor and get in some good practice. Grandma always loved her casino and dance show weekends with Marianne and Michael.

While they were gone, I regained energy that I didn't even know I had lost. I remember a few weekends where I just slept for 12 hours every day that Grandma was with my aunt. Knowing that Grandma was safe, knowing that I didn't have to jump up for every little sound while I was sleeping, knowing that I did not have to make breakfast…all of it allowed me to sleep so soundly that I'm sure I never moved at all!

The bottom line is this: you cannot give quality care to someone else without first taking care of yourself. In order to keep your mental sanity, you need a break. If you don't have friends, family, or neighbors who can take care of your loved one for a couple of hours, put a sign up at your local community college. Students always need some extra cash, a free dinner, or elder care work experience. Students going into healthcare are going to have more practical knowledge of the healthcare issues at hand and will be happy to use their newly gained health observation skills in real life!

Here are some ideas for wording that you might want to use on your **Help Wanted** sign.

Remember to post it on job boards at your local community college and nearby nail or beauty salons.

<u>Caring Help Wanted for Elderly Loved One</u>

- In-home
- Variable hours to fit your schedule
- Gain experience working with senior populations
- 1-3 hours preferable
- Play board games and card games
- Flexible

Ideal candidates:

- Students going into a healthcare field
- Caring individuals
- Patient
- Dependable

Contact: (First Name)....(phone or e-mail)

About the Author

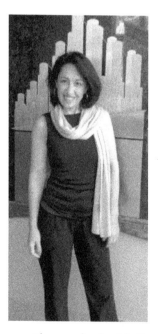

Lisa Santiago says that she has professional Attention Deficit Disorder because as soon as she can do a job easily, she's bored and moves on to something new. She's had many fun jobs including being a waitress, a sales associate for fine jewelry, and even a collections agent!

After earning her BA and MA, she spent the next decade working as an academic and personal advisor. She worked with first-generation college students, NCAA athletes, international students, and medical students. Earning an ED.S. in Higher Education

Administration with a focus on Counseling and Interdisciplinary Studies opened doors to another decade of guiding and serving people in ways she had never imagined.

Currently, Lisa works as a college professor - helping students apply their new knowledge rather than just memorize a bunch of facts. As a certified Life Coach, she works with a handful of select clients - helping them reach their personal and professional goals. She is also a certified Zumba instructor - teaching dance classes weekly. As her schedule allows, she enjoys giving presentations at educational and professional conferences across the US.

Friends have told her, "You would go further in life if you would focus on one thing." To this, Lisa says, *"I don't know everything, but this I know for sure: No person is just one thing. We all have a rainbow of gifts and life experiences to share with those around us. I want to use those gifts to make the world a better place. I cannot ignore all of my colors. If I did, I would get depressed and die, and I'm not ready for that just yet."*

Future plans include *Tips for Caregivers Volumes II and III*. These books will follow the progression of Alzheimer's disease - providing tips on how to cope as physical and mental health needs change for both the loved one and the caregiver.

Keep up with Lisa on her Facebook page dedicated to this topic: Alzheimers Help for the Caregiver. https://www.facebook.com/sadness2smiles/

You can also reach her via e-mail at:

alz.care.santiago@gmail.com

Easy-to-find Online References

Flett-Giordano, Ann and Ranberg, Chuck. "Give Him the Chair." *Frasier*. Season 1, Episode 19, 17 Mar. 1994, www.youtube.com/watch?v=xwNxt6aWVZ0

This powerful episode helps to give caregivers a better understanding of the value of personal items when an elderly loved one must move in to a new home. On YouTube, you can watch a clip of an informative and touching monologue by Marty in this *Frasier* episode, uploaded by alpineinc1, 5 February 2018.

History.com. "Rosie the Riveter." *History.com*, A&E Television Networks, 23 Apr. 2010, www.history.com/topics/world-war-ii/rosie-the-riveter

This link provides both text and videos detailing the history of this iconic image which was designed to recruit women into the workforce during World War II.

Indie, Movieclips. "Sundance Film Festival (2014) - *Alive Inside: A Story Of Music & Memory Featurette - Documentary HD.*" YouTube, 7 Jan. 2014, www.youtube.com/watch?v=8HLEr-zP3fc

This link provides a short clip of this documentary which helps us see the power of music in helping Alzheimer's and dementia patients recall memories. You can request the full DVD, for free, from any public library. The full documentary, directed by Michael Rossato-Bennett is 1 hour and 39 minutes long.

Reeltimeimages, *"Untangling Alzheimer's – Trailer."* YouTube, 14 Feb. 2014, https://www.youtube.com/watch?v=UA6vH6Hub6A

This link provides a short clip of this 2013 Netflix documentary which follows David Suzuki's quest to find answers to why Alzheimer's is such a mystery. In his quest he meets doctors and patients who are exploring and testing some of the newest treatments. The full documentary, directed by R. Verdecchia, is only 44 minutes long and explains some of the connections between Alzheimer's disease and diet.

TED. *"How to Make Stress Your Friend | Kelly McGonigal."*, YouTube, 4 Sept. 2013, www.youtube.com/watch?v=RcGyVTAoXEU

In this short Ted talk, you'll hear Stanford researcher Kelly McGonigal explain her research suggesting that your beliefs about stress, and your social connections, are the secret keys to your long-term health and happiness.

Unkrich, Lee and Adrian Molina, directors. Coco. *Coco*, Disney-Pixar, 2017, https://movies.disney.com/coco

This link takes you directly to the Disney web page for this film. It is an Academy Award-winning animated film focused on honoring ancestors on the Day of the Dead. Near the end of this film, there is a powerful scene where the grandson begins to sing to his great-grandma. The song, from her childhood, helps her recall powerful and happy memories that were about to disappear forever. You can request the full DVD, for free, from any public library. This film is 1 hour and 45 minutes long.

Wahls, Terry. " Start Here." *Getting Started on The Wahls Protocol*. Dr. Wahls, MD & Author, 7 Mar. 2019, https://terrywahls.com/start/

This website is written by Dr. Wahls. It includes a video link to the TEDx lecture that I saw in Iowa City, IA titled *"Minding your mitochondria."* This website includes links to additional current resources as well as data on Dr. Wahls' current and continued research.

CPSIA information can be obtained
at www.ICGtesting.com
Printed in the USA
BVHW080249130220
572225BV00001B/35